professional authority, or to draw attention away from problems caused by overall NHS funding limitations.

Against this background and the information in and questions posed by *A First Class Service* the objective of this report is to clarify the concepts and issues underlying national debate on health care quality. It offers a critical look at the claims made by proponents of quality management techniques. It also considers aspects of politicians', professional leaders' and managers' abilities to address the challenges of quality improvement.

The analysis presented draws in part on work conducted by the author while at the Audit Commission in mid 1990s (which provided the basis of a 1994 Commission note to the NHS Policy Board on quality management and the starting point for *Dear to Our Hearts?* [3] - a study on commissioning better services for the prevention and treatment of coronary heart disease) together with more recent qualitative research undertaken on behalf of the Fund.

The rise of quality management on the agenda of not only the NHS but many other public and private sector organisations has been driven by a combination of powerful historical forces associated with economic development, demographic change and increasing global competition (Box 1). To the extent that quality management techniques were originally developed to enable commercial firms improve their sectional sales and profits, there is a danger that the naive pursuit of 'better quality' in organisations like NHS Trusts could at worst draw attention away from the most important human goals that the health and social services exist to pursue. But this is not to say that more effective health and social care processes cannot be achieved through disciplined, well informed and intelligent application of health care quality management.

Although the latter may prove difficult to apply well, they have the potential to deliver important benefits in terms of lives saved and suffering and disability reduced. Everyone involved in care provision should therefore work to understand the lessons that quality management has to offer, without losing sight of the fundamental objectives which originally underpinned the establishment of the NHS, and professionalism in health care.

Box 1 - Forces driving health sector change and the rise of quality management on the NHS' agenda

Factors associated with recent shifts in the way health care systems are funded and managed include:

- **continuing national and international demographic transition,** resulting in population ageing in countries like Britain and rapid population increases in poorer nations. Medical and allied interventions can contribute to changes in the health status of populations, although normally economic and allied influences such as better food, education. housing and sanitation are the most important factors. As health and health and social care needs alter, so health services have to change;

- **intensified global economic competition,** associated with the above. This has put new pressures on countries like Britain to improve the productivity of its people and industries, and to maximise the value derived from all types of welfare expenditure;

- **raised consumer expectations, and greater questioning of traditional professional authority.** People are increasingly unwilling to be passive, unquestioning, users of health services, and more likely to demand information and care sensitive to their personal needs. This is in part a function of small family sizes linked with greater wealth, and increased sensitivity to risks to each individual's survival;

- **new patterns of professional training and workforce expectation,** generating in part demands for a more supportive environment and better cross agency co-ordination;

- **the application by Governments of competition policies and modern management techniques to traditionally autonomous areas of professional activity;** and

- **technical advances in medicine, coupled with an improved understanding of the social determinates of health and illness.** This has led to an environment in which it is increasingly possible to generate relatively small additional health gains through further large scale spending on 'high tech' medicine, while at the same time the health opportunity costs of failing to invest in other parts of the community infrastructure are becoming more visible than was in the past the case.

CONTENTS

ABOUT THE AUTHOR

David Taylor is a former King's Fund Fellow and Associate Director of the Audit Commission. He is currently Director of Health Affairs at GJW Government Relations. He is also visiting Professor of Health and Medicines Policy at the School of Pharmacy, University of London, and an external Professor of the Welsh Institute for Health and Social Care. The views expressed in this paper are those of the author.

1. INTRODUCTION

The 1997 White Paper *The New NHS: Modern, Dependable* [1] promised to put quality at the heart of the health service. The innovations it announced included:

- the formation of a National Institute of Clinical Excellence, to promote at national level (in England) work on clinical and cost effectiveness, and to draw up and disseminate guidelines;

- a Commission for Health Improvement to support and oversee the quality of clinical services at the local level;

- evidence based National Service Frameworks to help ensure 'consistent access to services and care quality';

- a new system of clinical governance in NHS Trusts, backed by statutory provisions and designed to 'put quality on the agenda of every NHS Trust board'; and

- an annual survey of patients' experiences of NHS care.

More recently the consultative document *A First Class Service: Quality in the new NHS* [2] (published in July 1998) provided a fuller description of the changes planned. Much of the detail of these and similar reforms being introduced elsewhere in the United Kingdom is not yet fully determined. But what is already clear is that they mark a significant step forward in the management of the health service. *The New NHS* promises a more integrated, focused and vigorous approach to achieving consistently high standards, intended to facilitate the pursuit of *'quality in its broadest sense: doing the right things, at the right time, for the right people, and doing them right - first time.'*

However, many clinicians - and indeed health service users - are likely treat any politically lead pronouncement on 'health care quality' with a degree of caution. This is in part because much recent national policy and local activity relating to this topic has - despite its considerable scale and scope - been fragmented, and often marginalised from the mainstream of clinical and managerial activity. The NHS has been described by critics as suffering from 'chronic quality initiativitis', involving a (frequently politically induced) failure to concentrate on any one line of development long enough to generate good results. 'Quality' has to date been treated as a 'bolt-on' extra rather than as fundamental to the way treatment and care are provided.

Definitive evidence of the value derived from the one to two billion pounds of public money spent on NHS and allied quality programmes since the end of the 1980s has proved difficult to gather. Cynics may even regard 'quality' projects as Trojan horses used to undermine traditional

2. CONCEPTS OF QUALITY

As beauty lies in the eye of the beholder, so quality lies in the needs and expectations of the user. Employed in this way the term 'high quality' does not necessarily mean that something is finely crafted, technically superior, made of superlative materials, exceptionally durable, or supplied in the most exclusive or 'professional' manner. Rather it relates to whether or not a product or service gives the person using it the benefits he or she genuinely most desires, given their affordability and the limits of the available technologies. Although complicated in 'imperfect market' areas like health by the fact that service users often lack the information and on occasion the insight needed to allow them to understand how best to achieve what they most want, the essence of quality is that control over its definition and evaluation rests ultimately with the consumer.

Definitions of quality such as 'fitness for purpose' stress the relativistic nature of this concept. But awareness of the fact that different people may - depending on their past experiences and current circumstances - have different requirements should not lead providers to dismiss the idea of quality as 'merely subjective'. In the value systems of all market economy based societies informed consumer preference is sovereign, subject to basic moral restraints. The ability to meet it in an appropriate manner is an absolute requirement for the long term success of any enterprise, public or private.

If a high quality good or service is defined as one with the attributes desired by the well informed customer, then the term quality management refers to the sets of skills needed to supply such products. These encompass the abilities needed to:

- understand customers'/users' needs, and the relative priority to be given to each quality dimension;

- enable everyone involved in the production process to work together effectively and efficiently, and in ways which motivate them to use all their energies and knowledge in complementary rather than conflicting ways; and

- analyse empirically processes of production and supply, so that those involved can correct sources of error and be empowered to find progressively better ways achieving agreed goals.

When outlined in basic schemata such as those shown in **Figures 1 and 2** (see appendix, page 33) quality management may appear easy to achieve. Its advocates and practitioners frequently claim that the approaches they offer will generate dramatic cost savings and major service benefits. But not all organisations can in reality achieve such gains[4]. There are a variety of factors which may act as barriers to the effective application of quality management concepts. The paragraphs below outline some of the more important issues which exist in this context, particularly as applied to the field of health and social care.

2.1 Definitional confusion

In the health sector corporate and professional service providers (such as doctors, pharmacists and nurses) all tend to emphasise the value of the particular parts of the care process at the centre of their roles. Thus surgeons may stress the importance of access to operations such as coronary artery bypasses or knee replacements while physicians (and pharmaceutical companies) may be more aware of value of medicines. Doctors often strive for cures while many nurses and social workers may place greater emphasis on caring and coping.

Similarly service managers and various patient groups may also have differing - and competing - concepts of an optimal health service (**Figure 3**). Managers are likely to be especially conscious of budgetary restraints, and hence the importance of cost effectiveness and financial incentivisation. Like public health physicians, they are likely to be concerned with achieving what they perceive to be the greatest good for the greatest number. By contrast consumers and their advocates (including clinicians who act as patients' agents, as well as care providers) may understandably seek the most effective individual care, whatever its cost.

References to the need to improve 'quality' can therefore all too often serve as shots fired in political battles for legitimacy and the moral high ground, and so control of resources. As such they can sometimes confuse rather than inform attempts to understand how best to allocate available funds.

A related problem is the tendency many commentators have to define quality in partial terms, arbitrarily separating certain aspects of a service from others. Thus some talk about cost/price as an attribute distinct from quality, while others distinguish between volume and quality. And in certain publications quality and clinical effectiveness are used as synonymous terms, while in others quality is taken to refer to service characteristics other than clinical effectiveness.

For example, in *The New NHS* White Paper quality and efficiency are referred to as two distinct phenomena which together describe all facets of health care. Yet in the equivalent Scottish document (entitled *Designed to Care*) clinical effectiveness, efficiency, access, appropriateness and equity all lie outside the term 'quality'.

While such variations may be unimportant in themselves they betray an intellectual uncertainty which runs throughout much public discussion of quality related issues. This ultimately stems from the fact that there is no single body of quality management theory, based on a commonly agreed set of principles such as those lying at the heart of disciplines such as, say, market economics or organic chemistry. Rather, there is a wide collection of sometimes conflicting ideas and philosophical constructs derived from the applied work of pioneers such as Deming - see Box 2.

The use of comprehensive, multi-dimensional models such as those offered by Robert Maxwell[5,6] and Avedis Donebedian (**Figure 4**) can help to clarify what is meant by the term quality. Yet its evaluation and achievement demands inputs from a wide range of disciplines. A quality management framework will reveal the need for inputs from health economists, medical sociologists and health psychologists, alongside those of clinicians. But it cannot replace them, or determine their relative importance. Clinicians and managers with responsibilities for quality need extensive support to fulfil their roles well.

2.2 Measurement problems

It is often argued that those facets of a complex service such as health care which may be most important to consumers (such as, say, the provision of a sense of trust, sustained community support and dignity to people who are in fear or pain) are the most difficult to quantify, whereas those which are easy to measure may often be less important. It is also commonly observed that in managed organisations that which is measured gets done, while those things that cannot be empirically quantified are frequently neglected.

Such assumptions can and should be questioned - there is no compelling reason why committed managers, for example, should not use qualitative measures alongside quantitative indicators to monitor less tangible aspects of organisational or welfare system function. And a wide range of relatively sophisticated instruments has now been developed to measure clinical quality [7]. Nevertheless, there is in practice a clear danger that priorities and goals will become distorted by the simplistic use of the types of performance statistic often embedded in top-down, centrally driven, quality programmes.

Comparative reference data can of course be of value in circumstances such as those recently revealed in the case of paediatric cardiac surgery at the Bristol Royal Infirmary. But even figures such as mortality variations between hospitals or surgeons can be very difficult to interpret. This is in part due to confounding factors such as the actions that may be taken by some service providers to avoid poor outcomes, and problems associated with analysing statistics relating to small, variable, populations. (In the Bristol case it may also be observed that it was not necessarily a lack of formal data which perpetuated poor service quality. Rather, it appears to have been a lack of social relationships and personal attitudes necessary to ensure that a visible problem was addressed in an open, timely, manner.)

In the United States the use of comparative mortality data as a guide to health care quality and organisational excellence has been questioned[9], as

Box 2 - the quality pioneers

Before the mid nineteenth century most things were made by craftsmen. A considerable part of the delight of their products lies - like that of personal care and attention - in their individuality. But hand made goods are relatively costly. By contrast, mechanised production can offer consistency, along with reduced cost. However, even small variations in machine-made items can undermine their functional quality. Recognising this early twentieth century American investigators such as Frederick Taylor concluded that factory workers needed to be trained to work with great consistency on simple, repetitive, tasks. This led to charges that industrial management techniques were in danger of turning people in automatons.

In the inter-war period a new generation of US analysts took forward management thinking in two key directions. Elton Mayo observed paradoxical improvements in workplace performance when conditions (in the Hawthorne electric light factory) were changed to provide either more or less light. The 'Hawthorne effect' results from the fact that people respond positively to interest being taken in them, and to the stimulation provided by being part of what they believe to be an important, high status, exercise.

Walter Shewhart was a physicist and statistician employed at the Bell Telephone Company. He observed that variations in production processes could be either a random function of unknown in-built factors (which he termed 'common' causes) or due to external, 'special', causes (such as, say, a power cut). The value of this is that production defects due to common causes have statistically predictable characteristics which allow them to be analysed, and where necessary 'engineered out'. In circumstances where problems are due to special causes management interventions of a different type are required. Changing the production process itself would merely be 'tampering'.

In the era following World War II there have been several sets of new quality management pioneers, including:

- 'early' Americans such as W Edwards Deming and Joseph Juran, who made important contributions to the reconstruction of Japanese industry and subsequently were taken seriously in the US and elsewhere in the West;
- Japanese authorities such as Kaoru Ishikawa, Genichi Taguchi and Shigeo Shingo, who applied engineering expertise and statistical control concepts to production management, leading to methods such as quality circles, zero defect manufacturing, 'just in time' production and delivery, and total quality control (later termed TQM); and
- new generation Americans such as Philip Crosby and Tom Peters, who in building on the ideas of preceding commentators emphasised concepts such as (internal and external) customer focus, management leadership and personal quality management.

There are significant inconsistencies between the approaches advocated by different 'gurus', and the extent to which techniques developed to improve production in commercial settings like factories can be successfully applied to the professional delivery of care in life and death settings may be questioned. However, the health sector work of individuals such as Don Berwick[8] demonstrates that important service contributions can be made. It may be concluded that there are a number of core ideas common to all quality management strategies, but these must be applied in a manner tailored to particular cultures and task imperatives.

have 'league tables' and the simplistic employment of comparative audit and allied information in the UK.

The imbalanced use of one form of measure (for instance, short-term bio-medical outcomes) as opposed to another (such as longer-term gains in social functioning) may also serve to compound service distortions stemming from political and allied pressures. This danger can be related to suggestions that in Britain recent trends towards a narrowing of the definition of health care and a broadening of that of (charged) social support has in reality disadvantaged needy groups such as the elderly chronically ill, even while NHS service 'quality' might be said from a technical perspective to have improved.

There is an additional possibility that misunderstandings about the relative importance of process and outcome measures have served to inhibit progress. The purpose of health care is to deliver better health outcomes, albeit that the latter should arguably be taken to include a timely and accepted death rather than a painful, drawn-out struggle for limited amounts of extra time. But this is not to say that end point outcomes represent the most valuable measures of performance in every-day practice. This is not least because they often take a long period to become apparent. Frequently process measures can contribute more to improved care management, provided they are based on good research on what processes eventually produce the end results most desired by patients.

A number of those interviewed for this study reported that past failures to appreciate the importance of appropriate quality measurement approaches have acted as a barrier to service improvement. However, most also believed that such problems are becoming better understood by both NHS managers and clinicians. The introduction of well researched National Service Frameworks (the first two of which will relate to mental health care and coronary heart disease prevention and treatment) should in future provide a better basis from which to pursue local care improvements via techniques such as care pathway based audits.

2.3 Levels of quality

Another important dimension of service quality which is often ignored or not fully understood is illustrated in **Figure 5**. Health and social care quality can be analysed at three quite distinct levels[10]:

- **the system (or community) level.** This involves care provision for a total population and the overall processes of resource allocation and re-allocation via taxation and insurance systems needed to fund equitable levels of care for all. The legitimacy of the power needed for control at this level is politically based, and the historical mainstay of its administration has been through official bureaucracies;

- **the institutional (or managerial) level.** This is the level of the particular hospital or practice, serving a partial population. In much of the world the driving force and ultimate legitimacy of power exercised in this context is essentially competition or 'market' based - that is, it involves choice exercised on the part of service users or their agents as to which particular institution is selected to provide a given service; and

- **the individual (or professional) level.** This is most commonly focused on the interests of particular patients and driven by codes of ethics, personal - at heart moral - commitment, and peer group pressure. It is the level at which overt accountability is most often demanded, although even here it is usually difficult to test.

When working in the overall public interest political authority can promote good care and better health by directing resources to areas where greatest benefits can be derived, and by balancing the pursuit of sometimes conflicting quality dimensions - see Box 3. Managerially led quality initiatives have traditionally contributed most to efficiency and 'customer service' improvements, while professionally led quality has in the past concentrated more on achieving clinical effectiveness and personal aspects of care.

The recent development of health and allied services has in most countries been marked by ongoing interactions and conflicts between each of these domains. A central challenge for the future is to find effective ways of achieving greater coherence between care quality improvement interventions at all three levels.

2.4 Driving out fear or eliminating bad apples?

A central element in the theories of quality management practitioners such as Deming[11] relates to the importance of driving out fear from organisations. This is because a key intermediate goal of quality management for gurus in this school is the achievement of cultural changes leading to the creation of learning organisations. These are characterised by high levels of staff involvement and personal commitment - see **Figure 6** in the appendix.

There are good psychological reasons for accepting the validity of such approaches, as well as a significant body of observational evidence (dating back as far as Elton Mayo's inter-war findings on motivation at the Hawthorne Electric Light Company) indicative of their effectiveness in practice. Nevertheless, research conducted during the preparation of this report suggests that such thinking remains alien to many senior managers in Britain.

In what remains a strongly class-based and often short-term results oriented society there is an underlying belief that authoritarian - coercive

Box 3 - Conflicting quality dimensions?
Efficiency, effectiveness and equity

Most products and services have a wide variety of desirable characteristics. A common reason for quality management failures is that insufficient effort is made to prioritise the attainment of improvement goals, or to resolve conflicts between them. Examples relevant to the past performance of the NHS and other health care systems range from an over-concentration on environmental and support service standards rather than clinical outcomes, to a lack of clarity on issues relating to trade-offs between different quality dimensions.

One illustration of the latter relates to tensions in countries such as the US - and more recently the UK - between purchasing-side organisations concerned with maximising efficiency (so that within a given budget overall outcomes can be maximised) and provider-side organisations and individuals who emphasise that the effectiveness of care should be maximised in each individual case. The credibility and value in practice of health care quality management depends to a considerable extent on the skill with which the intellectual and allied communication challenges arising in this area are met.

In Britain there may also be clashes between the pursuit of greater equity (defined as equality in health status between population groups) and the quality goal of maximising the total volume of health gain generated by health care.

Health services may be of the most absolute benefit to those who are relatively well-placed in life. Those who because of environmental or other long term factors have the worst health may not be able to respond optimally to either health promotion or treatment. Hence although more even standards of health across all community groups may be thought an inherently desirable target, its attainment could logically require dis-investments in the health service relative to other public or private provisions. Politically, however, this might not prove acceptable. This is not least because it could be judged unfair to those who contribute most to the NHS in terms of taxes, and thus inequitable as defined in commonly agreed terms of justice.

The most robust conclusion to draw from such observations is that quality management approaches in areas such health and health care for populations cannot effectively be applied without additional contributions from disciplines like health economics - which within the limits of the science available seeks to quantify and compare benefits as well as costs - or in isolation from political process. The latter is the ultimate arbiter of what is both possible and acceptable to the community in a given social situation.

11

rather co-operative, punitive rather than rewarding - management interventions are the most important keys to achieving improved performance. In contributing to the interviews on which this report is based one leading figure in public service management commented *'the lesson of history is that giving people a kick up the backside is normally the only way to get things done'*.

Some politically led discussion relating to the formation of the proposed new Commission for Health Improvement might be taken to reflect a pre-occupation with 'zero tolerance of failure' rather than an informed concern to help and empower NHS professionals working in difficult circumstances to cope better with the challenges they face. (The Commission was originally proposed before the last general election. The then shadow Secretary of State for Health Chris Smith, in a speech entitled *'Putting Quality at the Heart of Health Care'*, called for the creation of *'a national audit team to carry out a trouble-shooting role where there is a consistently failing provider'*.)

Taken too far 'liberal', non judgemental, approaches can of course be counter-productive. Some individuals are 'bad apples' who indulge in behaviours which should not be tolerated. Staff who abuse vulnerable children and adults in institutional care are an obvious case in point. So too are managers who abuse those over whom they have power. Fear of retribution may be necessary to keep such bullying in check. It may also be argued that certain forms of fear drive improved organisational performance, and are an essential part of the dynamics of both market competition and well run public systems - see Box 4.

Nevertheless, the logic of quality management requires attitudes which foster support rather than rejection or punishment, and the recognition of most people's desire to work well and contribute to the well-being of all around them. An inability on the part of the public in general and some politicians, clinicians and managers to accept this fact (and to invest in adequate quality management training and support for individuals designed to enable them confidently to give of their best) could yet prove one of the most potent and enduring barriers to effective quality improvement in the NHS, and many other UK organisations.

2.5 Top down or bottom up?

Following from the above, similar concerns relate to achieving an appropriate balance of top-down and bottom-up forces in quality improvement. The cultural transition sought in total quality management or business process re-engineering programmes is represented diagramatically in **Figure 7**. The inversion in relative status illustrated reflects a desire to put customer interests first, and to enable those people most immediately concerned with making and providing goods and services to do their jobs as well as possible.

Box 4 - Threat, fear, and the perceived need for improved quality.

Learning organisations need to eliminate counter-productive fear, and the defensive behaviours it induces. But at the same time individuals and groups free from any sense of threat may lack the will to improve existing products and services. A balance is needed. The model presented in this Box indicates how external threats can best be accommodated by quality improvement oriented organisations, and what forms of internally generated fear are most likely to harm performance.

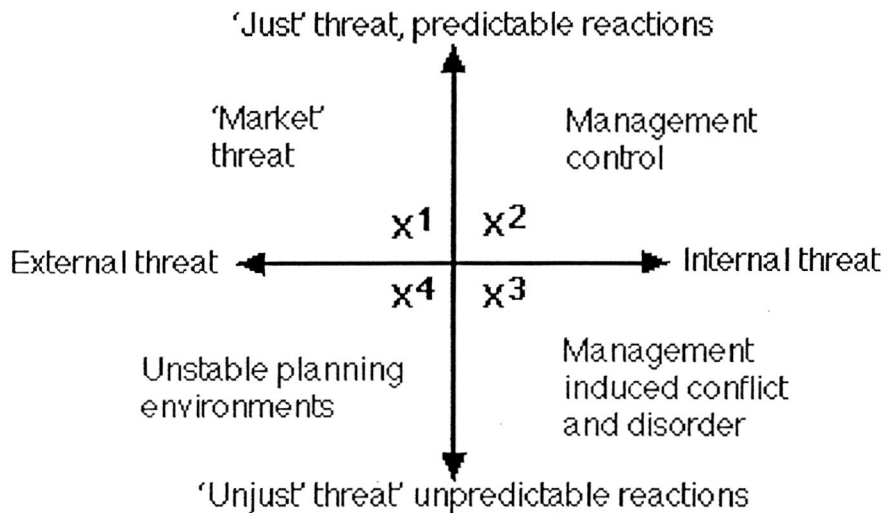

'Just' threat, predictable reactions

```
                    'Just' threat, predictable reactions
                                  ↑
        'Market'                           Management
        threat                             control

                        x¹  |  x²
External threat  ←──────────┼──────────→  Internal threat
                        x⁴  |  x³

        Unstable planning              Management
        environments                   induced conflict
                                       and disorder
                                  ↓
                'Unjust' threat' unpredictable reactions
```

The points marked x^{1-4} represent the following situations:

- x^1- **threat to the organisation and individuals stemming from external sources, accepted as just and predictable.** 'Perfect market' competition may threaten institutional survival and individual positions, as might the prospect of critical external audits from bodies such as the new CHI. If the members of the organisation can work together to mount an appropriate response then they have an opportunity to prosper. Fear can held in check, given a mutually supportive internal environment, and service quality stands to be improved.

- x^2 - **threat stemming from sources within the organisation, accepted as just and predictable.** 'Tough but fair' internal management can also be seen as vital for maintaining and improving quality. In health care informed consumer choice is difficult to achieve, and external inspectorates and commissioners may not be able to compensate for this. Strong internal management can, at least in part;

- x^3 - **threat stemming from within the organisation, experienced as unjust and unpredictable.** The 'bad boss/unfair employer' may use his or her power in an arbitrary, capricious, manner and deny others ownership of their work and the workplace. Such individuals are themselves 'bad apples', who serve to undermine the organisations they work in;

- x^4 - **externally originated threat, from what are seen as unjust and unpredictable sources.** Unpredictable, unjust threats - including, for instance, poorly planned re-organisations imposed on entire sectors - will not necessarily disrupt the working of internally cohesive, human value oriented, organisations. Indeed, such threats may even 'bring out the best' in people. But in time externally imposed changes which have no clear reason or pattern are likely to undermine morale, impair planning and generate counter-productive fear.

These are laudable ends. But on occasions they can be misinterpreted as requiring senior managers to surrender their duty to give strategic direction to their organisations, and take their proper share of responsibility for service standards. At the other extreme aggressive approaches to retaining top management's power during organisational development processes are also likely to be self defeating.

In health and social care organisations there is also a marked danger that attempts to introduce 'quality management' may only replace one power group at the pinnacle of perceived importance with another, rather than creating useful and appreciated changes in the way service users are served. For instance, it could be said that for most of the twentieth century teaching hospital consultants were the most important people in the health care world. In the 1980s they were to a degree displaced by senior Trust and other NHS managers, mainly from non-medical backgrounds. With the evolution of GP fundholding into locality commissioning there may be some risk that individual doctors and other staff in control of Primary Care Groups/Trusts could in future become seen as more important than those using the health service.

2.6 Paradoxical costs of 'better quality'

Advocates of quality improvement techniques often make considerable claims for their ability to reduce or eliminate financial the price of poor quality. Estimates of reductions of 30 to 40 per cent in total costs are frequently quoted. These may be gained by:

- reducing wastage associated with the rejection or re-working of inferior products, and compensation claims made in cases of negligence or other forms of poor service;

- reducing the costs of inspection, through integrating quality assurance and improvement concepts into normal working practices; and

- simplifying production processes and organisational structures by cutting out redundant stages and tasks. These inevitably build up over time if organisations fail to adapt to the introduction of new technologies and changes in their environments on a continuous basis.

There is no doubt that the gains obtainable from effective action in respect to the above can be very substantial, if not always as easy to demonstrate as participants in quality management activities initially anticipate. But at the same time the costs of improving quality, or attempting so to do, can be underestimated. Such costs may stem from:

- the high level of management input often needed to sustain reformed working practices, and constantly to maintain Hawthorne type effects on workforce productivity;

- the harm which can be caused to individuals and organisations through attempts to secure short-term economies which undermine trust and personal commitment; and

- the danger of increasing bureaucratisation as a result of paper based standard checking approaches, which can drive up inspection costs and employment in non-productive activities

Various commentators have pointed to the risks of 'form driving out substance' in health improvement programmes[12]. The ultimate hazard is that of the focus of quality management becoming in-turned, so that it becomes seen by those involved in it as an end in its own right rather than a means of producing better outcomes as reflected in measures like greater customer satisfaction and raised standards of public health.

2.7 Better management and stronger professionalism

The observations above indicate the scale of the challenges confronting those working to apply quality management techniques to the multi-faceted task of improving health and social care. They should not be taken to imply that striving to improve service performance through the application of such methods is either impossible, or impractical. But they do suggest that the intellectual and technical problems to be overcome in defining what better health and social care outcomes comprise, measuring their achievement, and enabling clinicians and others to perform better are much more complex than is sometimes implied.

At a political level, for instance, there has on occasions been an acceptance of approaches which have proved superficial. Such policies might in the short term have helped to generate favourable - if also transient - press reactions, and permitted positive sounding Parliamentary and media statements on 'getting to grips' with health and social care ills. Yet in the longer term they are likely to have achieved little save, perhaps, an undermining of professional morale and public trust. Genuinely worthwhile progress is only likely to be gained through a combination of sustained and thoughtful managerial and professional effort, focused on meeting the expressed and fully understood needs of service users.

3. PROGRESS IN THE NHS

Table 1 outlines the wide range of disparate quality initiatives introduced in the NHS from the mid 1980s onwards[13]. The fragmentation of effort required by and potentially counter-productive competition which has existed between these various approaches generated considerable criticism. Areas of concern identified by those who took part in interviews for this study, conducted both before and after the publication of *The New NHS*, include:

- the degree to which there has been a clear, trusted and commonly held set of values and purpose underlying NHS and allied welfare system developments;

- the extent of chief executive and other senior staff commitment to consistent quality management principles, and their ability to lead appropriate service improvement programmes;

- limitations in professional and other staff training in 'quality';

- inadequate clinical - and particularly medical - acceptance of the need for better management of care delivery processes;

- doubts about the value of audit programmes, and parallel to these related concerns about the recent emphasis on 'evidence based medicine';

- uncertainty as to the need for and role of service provider accreditation systems;

- uncertainty about the role and utility of user involvement initiatives and wider public communication activities undertaken by NHS bodies;

- lack of evidence as to the real value of commissioning, both at primary care and health authority levels;

- fears that the challenges of quality improvement in the area of primary and community care have not been addressed adequately; and

- concerns (expressed by individuals both working in the NHS and with responsibilities for its external inspection) that funding shortfalls affecting not only treatment but also management functions have not been adequately appreciated.

There is evidence that past centrally supported projects designed to introduce total quality management and allied techniques into NHS hospitals and allied organisations have not generated the benefits expected[14]. Issues relating to these criticisms and concerns are examined below.

Table 1 - NHS quality management initiatives

Initiative/technique	Description
Accreditation systems	Systematic approaches for assessing and verifying institutional and/or departmental, team or individual fitness to practice
Anticipated recovery pathways	Multidisciplinary patient journey based method for planning and monitoring treatment process
Audit (medical, clinical and organisational)	Cycle based approaches to identifying best - and current - practices and facilitating improvements amongst given groups of clinicians or managers
Benchmarking	Sets of techniques for comparing processes and outcomes between competitor organisations/groups
BS 5750/ISO 9000	A form of accreditation based on reviews of documentation on standard operating processes relating to each organisation's standards
Business process re-engineering	Radical review of organisational or clinical processes, implemented using total quality management techniques
Communications initiatives	Good communication with internal and external audiences is an integral part of quality management, although in the NHS 'communication' is still sometimes regarded as an 'add-on' activity
Complaints systems	Facilitation, analysis of and action to meet customer complaints is another integral component of TQM
Consumer surveys	Large numbers of variable quality patient and public surveys have been conducted in the NHS since 1990
Disease management	A term often used to refer to integrated single condition management programmes, associated with the US term managed care and pharmaceutical industry led programmes in Europe
Evidence based care/ NHS R&D programme	Initiatives such as the Cochrane Collaboration, the NHS Centre for Reviews and Dissemination and the NHS Health Technology Assessment programme all fall under this title. Techniques involved include meta-analytical reviews of research literature
External probity/value for money audit	Includes studies such as those conducted by the Audit Commission, which provide a national reports and a locally applied audit
Inspectorates	Organisations referred to under this title have included the now disbanded Health Advisory Service and the Mental Health Commission. The Commission for Health Improvement may, in replacing the CSAG, become 'a clinical Audit Commission'
Patients Charter	A set of monitored patient focused rights/care standards, first established in 1992.
Patient focus	An approach originally developed by US management consultants, which can be seen as a TQM variant. It concentrates on ensuring that patient's journeys through care are timely, convenient and otherwise of high standard .
Performance indicators and targets	Measures of activity and outcome used to assess performance and to promote enhanced care standards and cost effectiveness through comparison with national or local norms
Protocols and guidelines	Sets of treatment options and decision making criteria, reflecting best practice
Quality of life measurements	Instruments for assessing general or specific aspects of care outcome from a patient focused perspective. May be linked to the evaluation of treatment cost effectiveness.
Quality management assessment systems	Examples include the US Malcolm Baldrige award and the European Quality Award. They are forms of organisational audit
Risk management systems	An approach to quality based on the application of management tools designed to minimise the occurrence of events for which the organisation might be held legally or otherwise liable. Claims management is related to risk management; it is aimed at minimising costs after unwanted events have taken place
Total Quality Management (TQM)	Total quality management aims to involve everyone in an organisation in understanding external and internal customer needs and working together constructively to meet them, where possible using empirical measures of performance to inform their efforts. Continuous quality improvement (CQI) is a TQM variant

However, it is important not to exaggerate the faults of the NHS relative to other health care systems, and to be aware of the positive progress achieved within the NHS in the last two decades or so. There is no reason to believe that the problems encountered in applying quality management techniques to the delivery of comprehensive health and social care have been less in other European countries, or in the US. And for the overall amount of money spent on it the NHS already appears to deliver satisfactory outcomes in terms of overall population health and well-being, as compared with the data reported in other states.

Staff at all levels have worked hard in trying to take forward a great variety of projects, and most of those interviewed expressed positive views about prospects for the future. Many NHS staff members have in the past few years gained a sound awareness of quality improvement issues and techniques. Professional and management attitudes towards organisational change and the priority to be given to meeting patient defined needs have, in some important ways, already been fundamentally transformed.

This is evidenced by national level initiatives such as the involvement of the Medical Royal Colleges, the Royal College of Nursing and other professional bodies in health care quality improvement projects. Examples of these range from the organisation of workshops held jointly by the BMA and the National Association for Quality in Health Care through to the Royal Pharmaceutical Society's *Pharmacy in a New Age* programme[15]. The latter aimed to 're-engineer' aspects of pharmacy care.

It is also apparent in numerous local service improvement projects. Illustrations of these last range from investments in staff training in quality management (such as that provided through the Trent region SIGMA projects as well as through efforts made by individual hospitals like, say, the Hull Royal Infirmary) to sustained improvements in the co-ordination of community health and social care for chronically ill people. One example of progress in this field has been provided by a service improvement programme by the South Bedfordshire NHS Community Trust - see Box 5.

3.1 NHS values and service improvement

There is evidence of a general movement in NHS management and clinician attitudes to 'quality' since the early 1990s. The trend - which is mirrored in *A First Class Service's* emphasis on the fact that '*quality is not an add-on*' - is away from quality management being seen as an isolated function typically undertaken by displaced nurses managers or relatively low level bureaucrats. (One clinician summed up this view by saying '*quality management is the lady looking to see if the rubber plant has died'.*) It is towards continuous improvement being accepted as crucially relevant to that which all NHS managerial and clinical activity is intended to achieve.

18

Box 5 - Community care for people with stroke and allied disabilities in South Bedfordshire

Conditions such as stroke and allied forms of neurological damage or disorder can prove very disabling for those affected by them, and costly to the health service. As King's Fund research has highlighted, inadequate rehabilitative and supportive care in community settings can be a major cause of unnecessarily long hospital stays, and high hospital return and other institutional admission rates. Recent work by the Clinical Standards Advisory Group (CSAG) emphasised the opportunities for better service quality for people with stroke.

In the South Bedfordshire NHS Trust an improvement programme aimed at promoting better performance in this context began with a review of the available literature, followed by an extensive local survey of patient and carer experience of care and service users' requirements for achieving a raised quality of life. This revealed major shortcomings, and showed that measures commonly in use in hospital settings for determining patients' ability levels and support needs had little relevance to their functioning levels and service requirements in real life.

A new two stage assessment process was developed. This is aimed first at enabling care providers to satisfy patients' immediate needs when returning home from hospital, and subsequently at tailoring support to meet as optimally as possible the expectations and preferences of each individual in his or her particular setting. The monitoring system established indicates that improved outcomes have been achieved, while overall service costs have been reduced.

In some cases, however, the apparent integration of quality management posts into the mainstream of management activity may have been more the result of cost curbs than a genuine broadening of management objectives and ways of working. In this last context there is a degree of cynicism about the true objectives of people in senior managerial positions in health service and allied agencies.

A nurse employed in the care of elderly infirm patients in London summed this up when, after defining quality in terms of *'enabling everyone to understand (patients') needs more fully, and then being able to change to meet them'* she added *'but there are problems with management. From where we are you can easily see those whose ambition it is to climb, and those who want to do the best possible job for the sort of people you see here. The two things aren't the same and you don't have to guess who gets on the fastest'*. She then went on to outline some unwelcome service changes in her locality. Another senior nurse with considerable expertise in quality improvement commented *'everyone is just sick and tired of immoral management'*.

Such attitudes and fears may not be particularly unusual in any field. Nevertheless, the extent of concern which exists about the adequacy of NHS and social care (public) funding, and the barrier this could present to genuine quality improvement, should not be ignored. If attempts to economise become seen as the central purpose of quality programmes they are likely to fail.

The outcome of the Government's Comprehensive Spending Review may to a degree serve to put such concerns to rest. It provides for a 3.6 per cent annual growth in NHS 'real' resources over the life of the present Parliament, compared with the 3 per cent annual growth achieved by the last administration. But in the context of innovations such as the National Institute for Clinical Excellence there are some concerns that new demands for evidence of cost effectiveness could act as a 'fourth hurdle' in the process of introducing treatments into NHS usage. This could on occasion threaten rather than promote patient well-being. The UK's approach to change in areas such as, say, lowering cholesterol levels in people with coronary heart disease or introducing screening for type 2 (late onset) diabetes may already be considered to have been very conservative.

Similar considerations apply to debate about the reform of the welfare state generally. Beneficial progress is unlikely to be achieved in situations where those giving and receiving services do not believe that change is being proposed for legitimate purposes. Although the slogan 'quality is free' is true in competitive situations where those organisations which do not invest in service improvements will fail and so in effect pay for the success of their rivals, good quality health and social services are in many instances likely to more expensive - even if also better value for money - than poor ones. It is also a the case that the management and allied inputs required to support evidence based quality improvement programmes have themselves significant costs. The fact that there will be no new money to support the work of organisations such as NICE and the CHI raises some genuine questions as to what they will be able to achieve, at least in the short term.

Unobserved neglect is always the cheap option in situations where those in need can neither pay, nor seek redress for inadequate care and support. Such understandings underline the need for politicians at national level honestly to address health and social care funding and rationing issues. Attempting to appear to provide good - comprehensive - care with inadequate resources through devices such as devolving 'prioritisation' decisions to local health authorities or groups of family practitioners would be entirely inconsistent with concept of improving NHS quality as generally understood by the electorate, and service users.

3.2 Audit and accreditation

Audit of one form or another has long been the mainstay of professionally led quality improvement in health care. Audit cycles and quality improvement cycles encompass the same essential concept. Medical audit was in principle made compulsory within the NHS in 1989, at the time of the 'Working *for Patients'* reforms. It was also at around that time that the Audit Commission became responsible for the external audit of Health Authorities and Trusts in England and Wales. The Audit Commission designs and commissions both probity and value-for-money (VFM) audits.

Many health service managers were highly critical of medical audit in the early/mid 1990s. This was because of concerns about lack of access to its findings and the fact that it was often regarded as a part of continuing medical education and/or research, rather than as an integral aspect of overall care process management. NHS staff comments made at that time included:

- *'there is a veil of Masonic secrecy over the whole area';*

- *'it has underlined that there is one rule for the doctors and another for the rest of us';* and

- *'its been a nonsense in that a patient's treatment is not given by just one group'.*

It might be argued that a gradualist approach was necessary to achieve medical co-operation during the period of the 1990 changes. Nevertheless, the initial medical audit arrangements were unquestionably unsatisfactory, and in some instances at least helped perpetuate rather than alter unsatisfactory attitudes and practices.

The introduction of clinical audit from 1993 sought to address these limitations, although the extent to date of its effective contribution to patient care improvement is questionable. *'Whatever is said, the doctors who are not interested have just walked away'* is the way one observer summed up the situation early in 1998. An important challenge for the future NHS relates to the degree to which clinical governance can (together with contributions from agencies such as the Commission for Health Improvement) effectively drive the nation-wide application of clinical audit in a way which permits and encourages the local freedom and individual enterprise needed for achieving excellence, while also ensuring the reliable delivery of agreed national standards of care.

Topics to be considered in conjunction with the evolution of coherent national and local approaches to organisational and clinical audit include:

- the role of accreditation schemes;

- the development of evidence based medicine; and

- performance monitoring via the Patient's Charter and other indicator sets.

3.2.1 Accreditation

In the USA, which lacks an equivalent to the NHS management structure, accreditation via the Joint Commission for Accreditation of Healthcare Organisations (the JCAHO) has played an important role in attempts to establish standards across all dimensions of care quality. It has also contributed to structuring the US health care market, and may on occasions have served to inhibit cost competition.

Similar developments have taken place in countries such as Australia, Canada and Spain, while in the UK a number of related initiatives have been undertaken. The best known of these have been the King's Fund Organisational Audit Programme (now developing as an extended and more independent enterprise under the title of the Health Quality Service - HQS), the work of the Battle based Health Services Accreditation (HSA), and the process documentation focused British Standard 5750 (ISO 9000).

The DoH/NHS Executive approach towards accreditation in England has appeared largely unsupportive, despite repeated investments in its evaluation and the emergence of more positive attitudes in Scotland, Wales and many other states. Possible reasons for this include:

• fears of undue - and costly - bureaucratisation and of creating an excessive focus on (potentially costly) structural and procedural aspects of quality, as against the flexibility needed to achieve improved health outcomes despite on-going resource limitations; and

• uncertainties as to the need for both accreditation systems and the performance management structures already existing in the English NHS structure.

However, a more unified approach to independently provided accreditation currently has been created through the formation of the Health Quality Service. And the effective integration of the work of bodies such as the National Centre for Clinical Audit, the DoH funded National Guidelines and Professional Audit programmes, and the work of the Clinical Standards Advisory Group (CSAG) into the new NICE/CHI format should create a more streamlined and co-ordinated research, development and monitoring system on the public sector side.

A First Class Service suggests that the CHI will develop into the clinical equivalent of the Audit Commission, or perhaps a health care Ofsted. (The latter option is reportedly preferred by some advisors outside the DoH.) Key questions for the future relate to how the Audit Commission and the CHI will work together, and appropriately share the limited resources available for NHS external audit. In addition, there are significant technical challenges still to be overcome in developing a national audit programme capable of driving continuous improvement in clinical quality, rather than merely offering a 'tick box' approach to identifying alleged inadequacies.

3.2.2 Evidence based medicine

Evidence based approaches to enhancing clinical effectiveness have for some time been firmly endorsed by bodies such as the DoH and the NHS

Executive. In additional to programmes such as those run via (in England) by the NHS R&D Health Technology Assessment Programme, the Cochrane Collaboration and the NHS Centre for Reviews and Dissemination there a number of examples of Health Authorities (for instance, North Yorkshire[16]) and Trusts taking vigorous action to move their commissioning activities and care delivery priorities on to a firmer evidence base. This in part allows them to act as better customers for health service research agencies.

Such progress has much to recommend it, not least in as much as it promises to ensure that the standard setting at the heart of audit is soundly based. Yet there are also limits to the value of evidence based approaches. One of the most important is that they can encourage the ill-founded belief that a lack of formal evidence in itself 'proves' that a given intervention should not be provided. Concerns expressed during recent interviews with NHS professionals and care users relate to:

- the danger of an ongoing duplication of analytical effort in research institutes and public health departments. (This is, however, a problem that the National Institute of Clinical Excellence should help to resolve at the national level);

- corresponding failures to put sufficient effort into supporting the local implementation of clinical policies and desired practice changes; and

- limitations in the primary research available, and the danger of diverting health service activities away from 'softer' but in reality important aspects of care which cannot be easily subjected to randomised controlled trials. The hazards of inappropriate generalisation and spurious rationalisation were also raised. For example, it is sometimes falsely assumed that data on average service provision levels offer insight into the risk of inappropriate care being given or appropriate care being withheld.

One possible conclusion to draw is that the further raising of NHS quality will in time demand radical review of NHS public health 'medicine'. Control of this essentially generalist function at the heart of standard setting and implementing local level health service plans by one largely autonomous professional group cannot be considered in the public interest, or consistent with quality management principles.

Risks of distorting treatment and care priorities and activities may also be generated by quality improvement programmes based on numerical targets and performance indicators. Top-down goal setting and achievement monitoring is popularly considered a vital part of effective management, and the introduction of such measures may gain mass media plaudits. But the danger of imposing targets on workforces undertaking complex, specialised, tasks is that important but hard to quantify contributions will be driven out in favour of more tangible ends.

This central message of quality management 'gurus' such as Deming is often ignored by the proponents of mechanistic and/or simplistic approaches to activities such as internal and external audit. And powerful though the 'naming and shaming' use of devices such as league tables may at first seem to be (particularly when combined with financial reward and punishment systems) administrations use them at their peril. The available evidence suggests that in the longer term they risk not only alienating and de-motivating many people working in the organisations they are seeking to improve, but also creating a 'Soviet economy' of management information. Workers usually find ways of undermining or subverting the application of performance measures they consider to be inappropriate or unjust.

3.3 Communication and consumer participation

Good communication practice lies at the centre of good quality management, and of the role of the successful chief executive and his or her management team in any organisation. Effective communication plays an essential part in allowing external service user preferences to be understood, and in enabling internal provider groups to work together productively. It also helps to shape consumer expectations, and to permit patients and others to use services in an optimal manner. Hence communication programmes can constructively influence the definition of good service quality, and aid its delivery at all levels (**Figure 8**).

But this is not always adequately realised in public - or indeed private - service environments. This in part because in the past communication initiatives have been mounted in isolation from other attempts to enhance quality management. Individuals identified as communication post holders have often appeared to occupy relatively unimportant places in NHS agencies. In handling crises about topics such as, say, hospital closures or mental health care 'scandals' they sometimes seem over-defensive, rather than prepared and able to listen to local voices and respond seriously and honestly to the concerns expressed. One individual in a senior health service communications position commented *'the truth is we have been in the broadcasting business, not reception'*.

There are a variety of factors underlying such problems. They include:

- politically imposed controls, and fears of punitive responses to perceived errors of judgement. These can inhibit pro-active, fact based, approaches to improving patient and public understanding of health and social care issues. Pressure for political control of detailed aspects of NHS activity accounts for some of the special quality management and allied communication challenges facing those working in the service;

- failures to invest adequately in the research and managerial staff capacities needed to sustain good communications; and

24

- lack of commitment to act in accordance with overt NHS principles and values, even when patients are able to feed back experiences of service inadequacies. This may often be a consequence of resource limitations. But insensitivity to service users' needs can also stem from causes such as an inability to accept the legitimacy of patient demands for control over care and treatment processes. When asked about the apparent failure of NHS providers to respond to patients' concerns about poor pain control following day surgery and other operations a medically qualified respondent argued against greater use of approaches such as patient controlled analgesia. His grounds were that *'pain is notoriously subjective'.*

Increases in the numbers of patient surveys conducted in the late 1980s and early 1990s, and more recently the use of techniques such as patient or citizen's juries, illustrate some of the strengths and weaknesses of NHS progress in the communications and quality management field. On one hand many people working in the NHS have put considerable effort into organising such activities, and have with good faith attempted to translate their findings into practice. But on the other the results of such exercises have often been superficial, or already known, while the process of actually achieving better care has in many cases been frustratingly slow.

For instance, patients' concerns about and dislike of mixed sex wards have been well known for many years, but often not acted upon. Similar points can be made in relation to inadequate pain management after day surgery. To be of optimum value the national survey of patient and service user experiences of NHS care to be introduced as part of the new quality arrangements will need to be specified in a manner which takes into full account existing knowledge, and designed to generate fresh rather than recycled insights into consumer requirements. This may demand qualitative rather than quantitative research.

Continuous quality improvement demands a high level of intellectual input, coupled with uncompromising personal and organisational integrity. The simplistic application of management instruments of any type, from audit guides to patient surveys to the organisation of public meetings, may give an impression of action and positive service user consultation. Yet valued organisational and personal change is likely to require a much more reflective approach. It should clearly differentiate between research activities and care process standard setting and monitoring, and be based on a real respect for the fundamental needs and aspirations of those involved in providing and receiving care.

3.4 Commissioning better services

The 1990 NHS reforms introduced - as a key aspect of the new 'market' structure favoured by the then Government - a clear division between the Health Authorities responsible for purchasing or commissioning care for populations and the NHS Trusts and other agencies responsible for providing it. They also created GP fundholding. This, despite the controversy surrounding it, created a new motor of local service improvement.

In the main the developments outlined in 'The New NHS' build on logically these arrangements, and on the thinking contained in previous White Papers such as 'A Service with Ambitions[17]'. The terminology of the internal market has gone, and with it the concept of individual practice fundholding. Nevertheless, Health Authorities are to retain a separate commissioning status, working with Primary Care Groups and NHS Trusts to plan and facilitate the achievement of health gains.

Given the associated proposals aimed at strengthening NHS quality management and monitoring its performance within a new multi-dimensional framework (Box 6) there is substantive reason to believe that positive progress will result. However, new structures cannot in themselves provide solutions to challenges which stem from basic aspects of care processes and patient/professional relationships. Nor are desired changes likely if all the factors likely to prevent them happening are not honestly addressed.

In the context of care commissioning the challenges identified in this and other studies (including the Audit Commission report 'Dear to our Hearts?') include:

- limited data on patterns of service provision and delivery;

- limited data on service users' varying needs and priorities;

- limited evidence on the efficacy and effectiveness of preventive, therapeutic and rehabilitative interventions, particularly within differing population sub-groups;

- lack of clear criteria for making resource allocation decisions, and potential conflicts between the priorities of national level decision makers and locally based groups; and

- the difficulties inherent in improving the co-ordination of primary, secondary and tertiary health care and complementary social care and support, and in promoting changes in clinical practice.

Such barriers to care improvement will remain significant throughout the foreseeable future, particularly if the resources available for quality management training and projects at district and locality levels are not increased. The magnitude of the effort needed simply to support the set up of the Primary Care Groups in England and similar bodies elsewhere in the UK should not be underestimated. Challenges range from determining the scope of the decision making to be taken by PCGs to working out how professionals operating in such groups will be able to balance respect for individual patient requirements with pressures to comply with budgetary limits, and locally agreed policies.

Despite recent investments made by bodies such as the Royal College of General Practitioners in attempts to define 'quality' in primary care, many practical questions remain to be resolved. Generating effective solutions is likely to require considerable managerial, as well as professional, effort. In the light of this several of the managers and quality improvement oriented professionals interviewed believe that political rhetoric about 'cutting the costs of health service bureaucracy' threatens to undermine the viability of the new proposals. It can be insulting to NHS management staff, and may imply a failure fully to grasp the type of organisational developments needed to achieve more patient focused care processes.

In the area of primary care in particular there has arguably been a long term political level deficit of understanding relating to the nature of the challenges facing family practitioners, and the varying needs of the consumer groups using their services. Management attitudes developed in the context of hospital care provision are of little relevance to meeting the challenge of improving primary care. It remains to be seen how effective the approaches currently being introduced will be in promoting better NHS primary care quality without alienating service users such as better-off members of the population accustomed to personal care from their general medical practitioners.

4. CONCLUSIONS- CONTINUING THE IMPROVEMENT PROCESS

Quality management is not simply a passing fad in the NHS, reflecting a transient interest in an 'arcane Japanese cult'. Successive Governments have emphasised that the creation of mechanisms for achieving better ongoing clinical and support service improvement is a central component of national policy. All the main health care professions have also publicly accepted that care process improvement issues are of vital importance, and that a central duty of professional bodies is not only to maintain but progressively to better care standards.

Initiatives such as the health care and professional process re-engineering pilot projects recently undertaken in the Leicester Royal Infirmary and King's College Hospital in London (and in organisations not in receipt of special funding, like the Gloucester Royal Infirmary and the South Bedfordshire NHS Community Trust) have demonstrated that significant NHS service enhancements can be achieved. Roll-out programmes based on such experiences promise better care throughout the country, for less financial input than that required in pioneer sites. Whatever the weaknesses NHS approaches to quality may in the past have had, the service is now relatively well placed to move forward in its quest to provide good, affordable, care for all.

However, optimism should not be permitted to obscure the conceptual issues outlined in this report, and the remaining barriers to success. Notwithstanding international evidence of their capacity to improve health outcomes[18,19], quality management approaches have on some occasions been over-sold. Financial savings and service enhancements can be more difficult to realise than enthusiasts suggest. The maintenance of service gains often requires sustained investment of management effort, not least to guard against creating unduly time-consuming and unproductive paper based monitoring procedures. Further, no quality checking process can obviate the need for intelligence, flexibility and a willingness both to innovate and take risks in uncertain circumstances. Real success demands much more than identifying and correcting failures.

4.1 Valuing patients and staff

Progress in quality management requires a coherent understanding of human motivation, and the psychological needs of those providing and receiving services. There is considerable evidence that people of all ages value a sense of control in their lives and over what is happening to them, even if they elect to let health care experts and carers whom they trust make decisions on their behalf. Helping people to cope well with illness and disability demands respect for each person's need for autonomy, dignity and self-esteem, even during terminal care.

A similar respect for staff members' personal needs in their working lives is not always apparent within the health and social care system. This may be reflected in (often politically and media driven) biases in managerial attention towards attempts to 'root out failure', rather than helping the great majority of NHS employees to work even more effectively.

One of the most important matters to be addressed in connection with the Commission for Health Improvement and clinical governance is the extent to which such arrangements will in practice lead to the establishment of a system of constructive, genuinely effective, professional support and service development. A weakness of the NHS in past years has been a tendency to rely on scandal and outrage as a motor of change, rather than the systematic pursuit of excellence. This has been particularly so in 'Cinderella' areas such as mental health and learning disabilities.

Other key issues raised by the policy proposals and questions contained in *A First Class Service* include:

- **the role of NICE in health promotion and public health.** A strong case exists for arguing that the National Institute's role should swiftly be extended to include the development of evidence based approaches to health risk reduction, early stage disease screening and other aspects of public health improvement. This may demand use of data other than that generated by randomised controlled trials. But if the NICE agenda is not extended in this direction there is a danger that its work will bias rather than improve the overall pattern of service provision;

- **the need for more innovative primary research into the social and psychological aspects of patients' and other service users' needs.** Despite work by organisations such as the College of Health on topics like the social functioning of older people waiting for and receiving surgery, there is still a marked lack of adequate information relating to NHS service users' qualitative care experiences, and highest priority personal needs. This problem may be solved through the introduction of the new annual survey of patient's NHS journeys. But if information shortfalls remain additional provisions (like, for example, a new NICE led confidential enquiry on the quality of care in the last year of life) will be needed;

- **the need for further understanding of the ways in which desired service improvements can best be promoted.** Although their findings are usually dressed in 'hard' language the real achievements of interventions such as, say, national VFM audits and inspections conducted by external agencies are in reality no more certain than those of apparently 'soft' activities such as health promotion. Questioning, creative and open ways of evaluating the impact of such audit programmes are required. More attention may well be needed to be given to tasks such as developing and supporting the use of effective self-help instruments for improving the performance of health care organisations, units and individual professionals;

- **the role which fully independent accreditation bodies ought to play in NHS quality improvement, and whether or not a greater separation between financial control and service standard protection should be introduced.** If, notwithstanding the introduction of (as yet unspecified) statutory quality responsibilities within the NHS structure and recent funding announcements, tensions between pressures for public service economy and the population's expectations of better services remain unresolved, further radical reform of the English system will be required;

- **appropriate medical authority.** Ill-judged attempts to undermine legitimate professional authority impair health care standards. Successful health care quality management empowers doctors, nurses, pharmacists and the other professionals they work with to do their jobs as well as possible, rather than placing them in a straight-jacket of regulation. However, there is also a need to guard against undue medical control in areas such as public health improvement and external clinical audit, and to ensure a proper balance of authority in organisations such as PCGs and PCTs. Accepting inappropriate arrangements as 'the price of progress' would undermine quality;

- **primary care development.** The proposals contained in *A First Class Service* do not address in depth the challenge of primary care quality improvement, upon which much of the overall NHS's performance ultimately hinges. This may in part be due to the political sensitivities surrounding recent negotiations on the formation of PCGs and PCTs. But it may also reflect some continuing lack of awareness of the scale of the supportive managerial and staff investments still required;

- **resourcing quality improvement.** Following on from the above, the need to put adequate financial resources into the activities undertaken by NICE, the CHI and other components of NHS management must also be recognised if desired service gains are to be realised. Despite comment in *A First Class Service* relating to the costs of poor quality, quality management is not free. It may in time be possible to rationalise certain disseminated research and public health functions. Further growth in the pharmaceutical budget might also - rightly or wrongly - prove to be a target for economies. But in the short term the case for spending new money on stronger quality management is itself strong;

- **promoting patient power.** Surveys and consumer representation on decision making bodies are no substitute for empowering individuals from all social classes to be able use professional services to optimal effect in the pursuit their personal health and related goals. All actors in the NHS and local government need fully to recognise this critical determinant of quality (and the fact that facilitating better self care lies at the heart of virtually all good health care) and work together to meet service users' information and health and social care control needs.

4.2 Professional opportunity, managerial facilitation and political responsibility

The new NHS reforms represent a step back from competition driven cost control and service improvement towards a more managerially focused, politically led, system. However, the Conservative Governments of the last twenty or so years also intended that the NHS should meet patient and population need through high standard care. Their use of White Paper titles such as 'Working for Patients' illustrated the nature of the challenge laid down to managers and professionals alike. New Labour's approach continues this thrust, albeit with enhanced emphasis on central standard setting, greater local service integration, and firmer management of clinical processes in both primary and hospital care settings.

A good case can be made in favour of this strategy. Yet political impositions alone cannot secure desired improvements in health and social care. Politicians do not directly provide services, and they and the healthy majority who vote for them are unlikely to have as full an understanding of - or concern for - the detailed needs of sick and distressed people as do clinicians who offer care on a daily basis. Indeed, competition for electoral advantage could on occasions have just as damaging impact on the NHS as ill-managed competition inside the service.

Hence although national and local politicians have important leadership responsibilities, the improvement of care quality remains critically dependant on professional good will, along with that of managers. Doctors, nurses, pharmacists and social workers ought to become increasingly able to work across traditional functional boundaries in order to achieve better co-ordinated patient care. This may well break down traditionally isolated professional identities, and in so doing threaten some traditional interests. Yet such developments will also offer new ways of defining professionalism in health care, with quality improvement skills becoming more closely integrated with clinical expertise.

Some professional representatives might see in this opportunities for reversing recent changes which have led to a greater role for general management in the health sector. But the most important concluding message to emphasise in relation to the pursuit of better health and health care is that it cannot be attained through any one 'supply side' group 'winning' against another. Rather, it demands better understanding and improved co-operation between all those involved in the provision of health and related social care services at the national (system), local (institutional) and individual care levels. The end-point goal is the generation of a shared political, managerial and professional commitment to understanding and striving whole-heartedly to inform and meet the varying needs of health service users, as they choose to define their priorities and goals during their lives and, ultimately, their deaths.

31

REFERENCES

1.   Cmnd 3807, 1997. *The new NHS: modern, dependable*. The Stationary Office, London.

2.   Department of Health, 1998. *A First Class Service: Quality in the new NHS*. The Department of Health, London.

3.   Audit Commission, 1995. *Dear to Our Hearts? Commissioning services for the treatment and prevention of coronary heart disease*. HMSO, London.

4.   Pollitt C., 1996. *Quality in Health Care* **5**: 104 - 110.

5.   Maxwell R., 1984. *British Medical Journal* **280**: 1470 - 1472.

6.   Maxwell R., 1992. *Quality in Health Care* **1**: 171 - 177.

7.   Brook R. H., McGlynn E. A. and Cleary P. D., 1996. *New England Journal of Medicine* **13**: 966 - 969.

8.   Berwick D. M., Godfrey A. B. and Roessner J., 1991. Curing Health Care. Jossey-Bass, Oxford.

9.   Blumenthal D. and Epstein A. M., 1996. *New England Journal of Medicine* **17**: 1328 - 1331.

10. Foster A., Ratchford D. and Taylor D. G., 1994. *Quality In Health Care* **3** (suppl): 16 -19.

11. Deming W. E., 1992. Out of the Crisis. Quality, Productivity and Competitive Position. Cambridge University Press, Cambridge.

12. Maxwell R., 1997. Personal communication.

13. Taylor D. G., 1996. *British Medical Journal* **312**: 626 - 629.

14. Centre for the Evaluation of Public Policy and Practice, 1994. Total quality management in the National Health Service: final report of an evaluation. CEPP/Brunel University, Uxbridge.

15. The Royal Pharmaceutical Society of Great Britain, 1997. Pharmacy in a New Age. RPSGB, London

16. North Yorkshire Health Authority, 1997. Clinical Effectiveness Discussion Document. NYHA, York.

17. Cmnd 3425, 1996. *The National Health Service: A Service with Ambitions*. The Stationary Office, London.

18. Laffel G. and Blumenthal D., 1989. *Journal of the American Medical Association* **20**: 2869 - 2873.

19. Dixon N., 1998. Personal communication.

APPENDIX

Figure 1 – The Audit Commission Quality Map, and the Audit Cycle

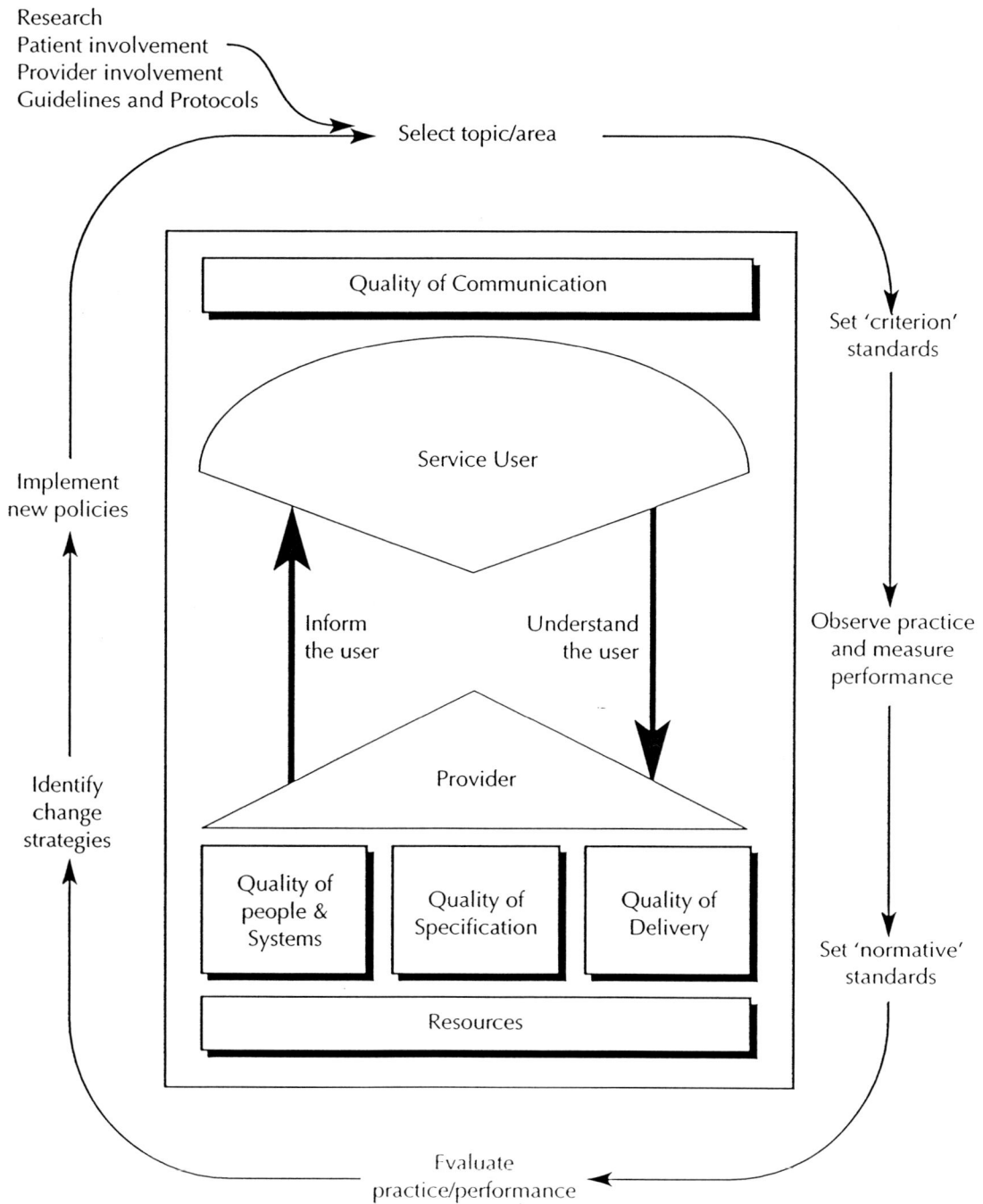

Research
Patient involvement
Provider involvement
Guidelines and Protocols

Select topic/area

Set 'criterion' standards

Quality of Communication

Service User

Implement new policies

Inform the user

Understand the user

Observe practice and measure performance

Provider

Identify change strategies

Quality of people & Systems

Quality of Specification

Quality of Delivery

Set 'normative' standards

Resources

Evaluate practice/performance

Figure 2 – The Malcolm Baldrige Quality Award Framework

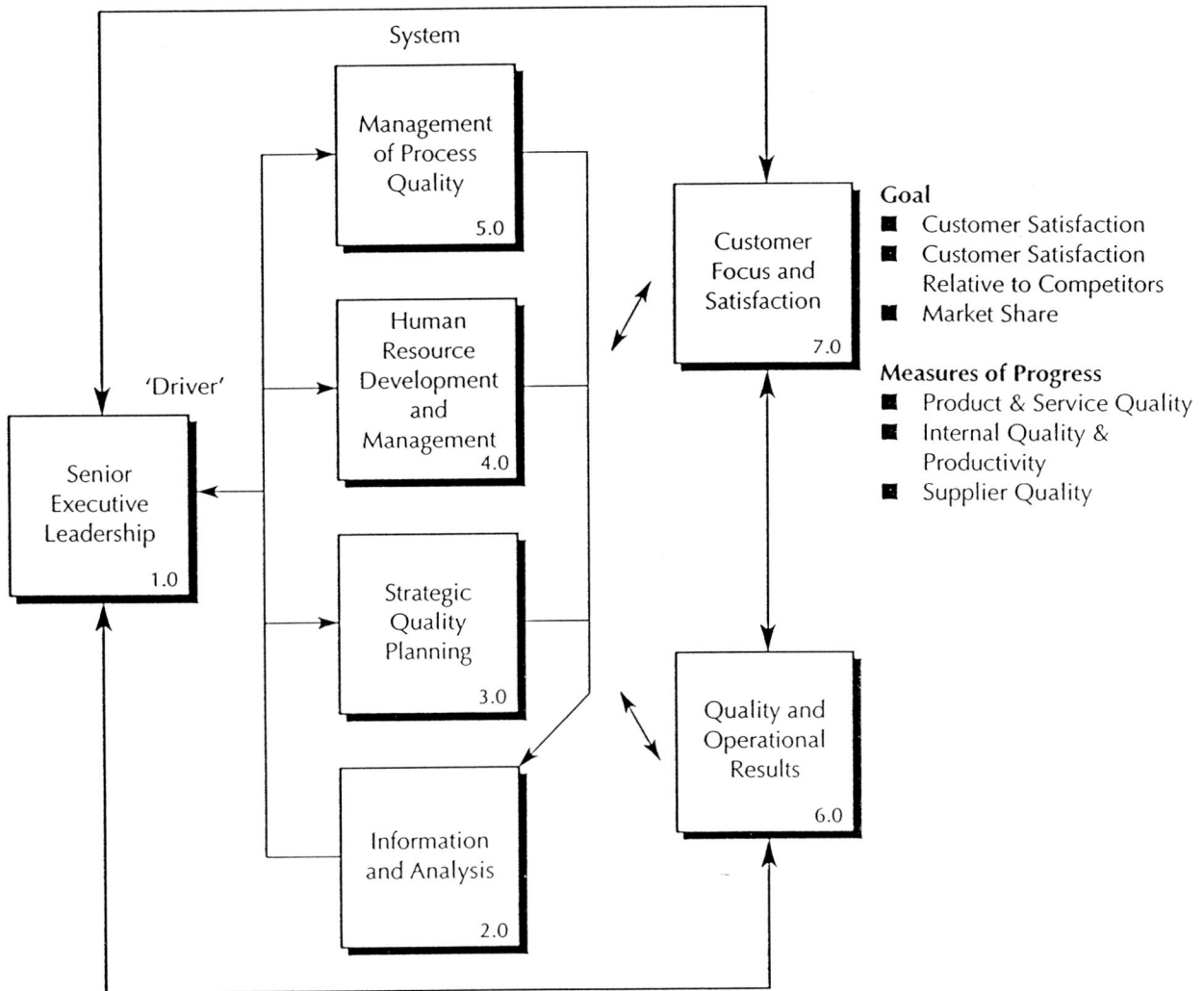

System

Management
of Process
Quality
5.0

Human
Resource
Development
and
Management
4.0

'Driver'

Strategic
Quality
Planning
3.0

Senior
Executive
Leadership
1.0

Information
and Analysis
2.0

Customer
Focus and
Satisfaction
7.0

Quality and
Operational
Results
6.0

Goal
- Customer Satisfaction
- Customer Satisfaction Relative to Competitors
- Market Share

Measures of Progress
- Product & Service Quality
- Internal Quality & Productivity
- Supplier Quality

Driver
Senior executive leadership creates the values, goals and systems, and guides the sustained pursuit of quality and performance objectives.

System
System comprises the sets of processes for meeting the company's quality and performance requirements

Measures of Progress
Measures of progress provide a results-orientated basis for channelling actions to delivering ever-improving customer value and company performance

Goal
The basic aim of the quality process is the delivery of ever-improving value to customers

Figure 3 – Quality Perspectives and Sectional Concerns

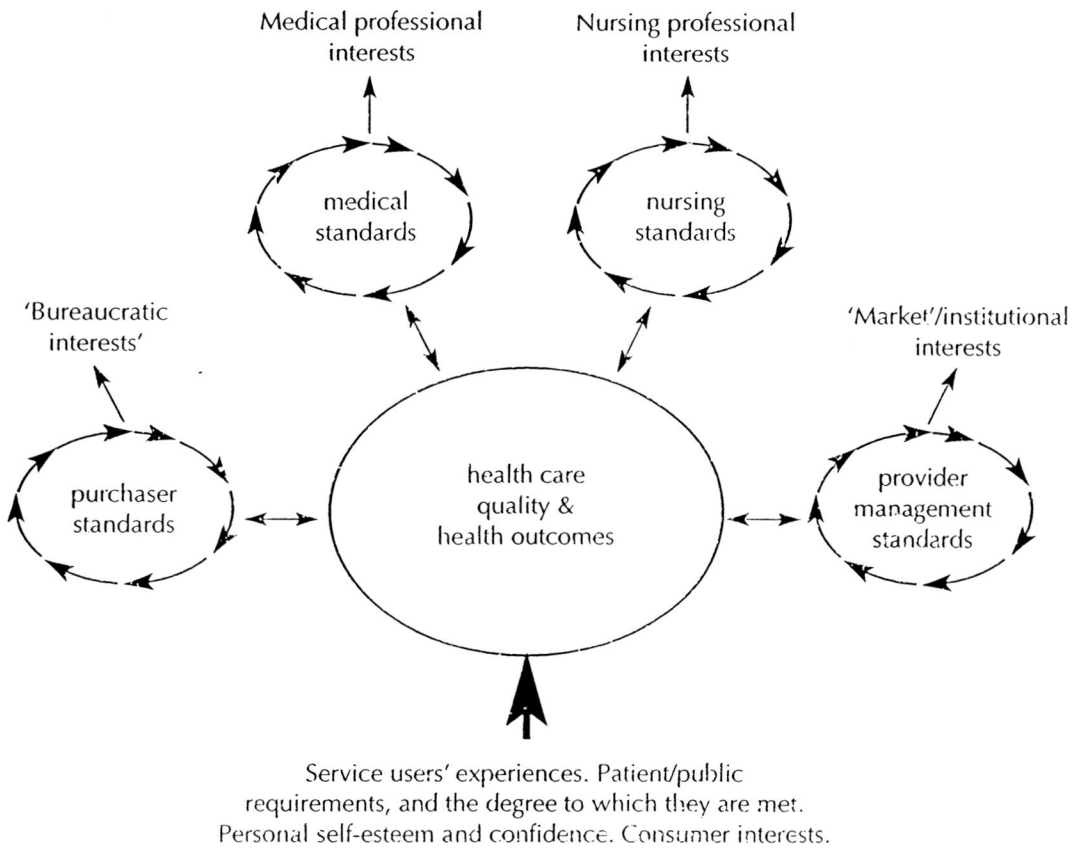

Medical professional interests

Nursing professional interests

medical standards

nursing standards

'Bureaucratic interests'

'Market'/institutional interests

purchaser standards

health care quality & health outcomes

provider management standards

Service users' experiences. Patient/public requirements, and the degree to which they are met. Personal self-esteem and confidence. Consumer interests.

B. The above model rests on the following definitions of quality:

Traditional quality:	Conveying prestige; a "quality" service can be seen as one which raises the self-esteem and confidence of the user (and its providers).
Scientific and professional quality:	Based on "expert" set standards and peer group values. Professionals internalise their collective norms and imperatives, expressing them in terms of their (moral) duties to patients.
Bureaucratic "management" quality:	Demands compliance with top-down set rules, impartially applied. Measurements of performance reliant on indicators approved by the internal hierarchy. Standards set by experts, but ultimately under political control. Legitimation via the ballot box or in communist/fascist societies the facts of social control and armed force.
Market "management" quality:	Derived from consumer willingness directly or indirectly to pay for a service or goods offered in a competitive market place. Cannot without extensive regulatory intervention maximise consumer well-being in imperfect market conditions, but may still be able robustly to protect general public interests.

Figure 4 – Dimensions of Service Quality

	Structure (resources)	Process (activities)	Outcome (results)
Effectiveness	Do staff qualifications conform with stated requirements?	Are best practice clinical guidelines and protocols adhered to?	
Acceptability	To what extent are facilities judged satisfactory by users?		Is the quality of life available to people with chronic conditions such as schizophrenia acceptable to them and the general community?
Efficiency			How does the cost per successful unit of treatment compare in one provider unit as opposed to another?
Access		What proportion of the total population in need of a treatment receives it, after how long?	
Equity		Is there bias in access between social groups, and is this judged fair by the community?	
Relevance	Do staff deployments match the patterns of expressed consumer need?		Do health gains resulting from existing patterns of care match those which could be generated by alternatives?

Figure 5 – Levels of Health Care Quality

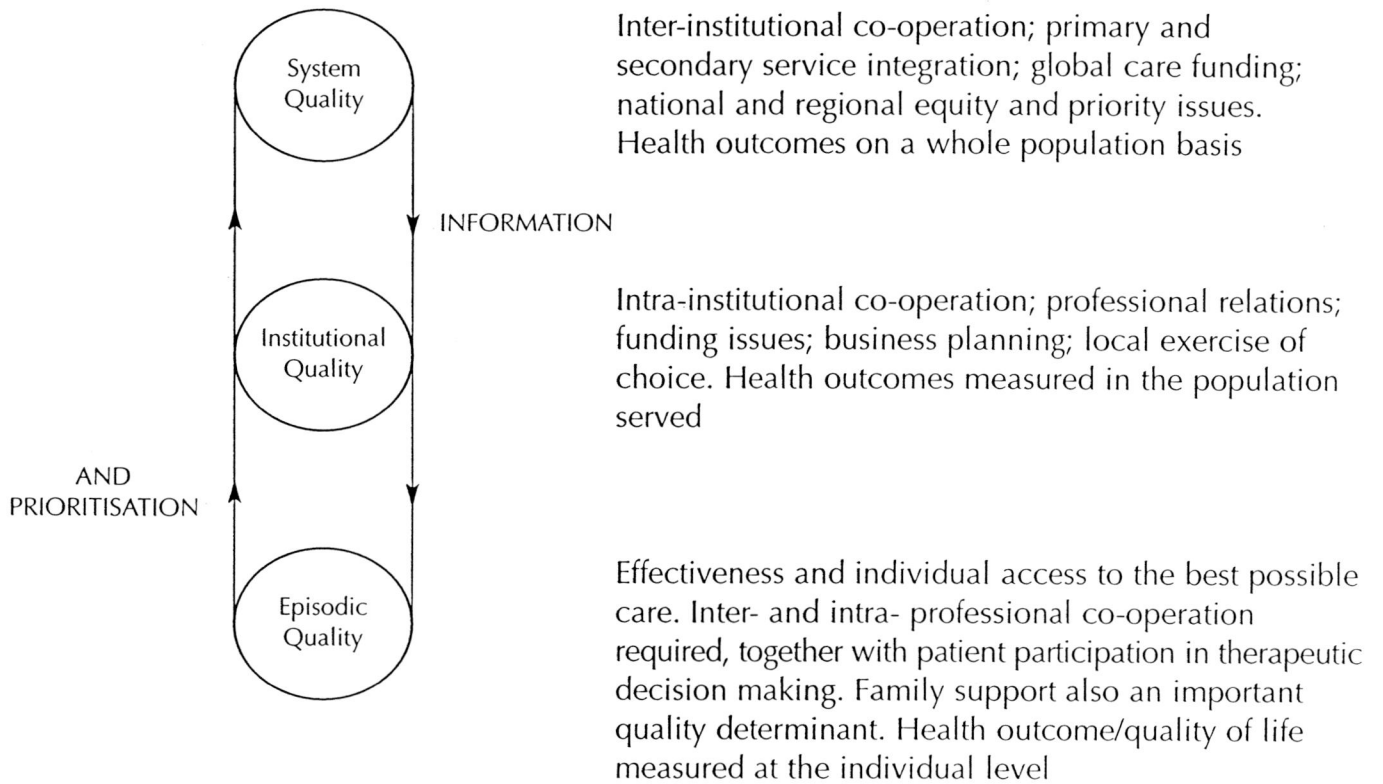

Inter-institutional co-operation; primary and secondary service integration; global care funding; national and regional equity and priority issues. Health outcomes on a whole population basis

INFORMATION

System Quality

Institutional Quality

Episodic Quality

AND PRIORITISATION

Intra-institutional co-operation; professional relations; funding issues; business planning; local exercise of choice. Health outcomes measured in the population served

Effectiveness and individual access to the best possible care. Inter- and intra- professional co-operation required, together with patient participation in therapeutic decision making. Family support also an important quality determinant. Health outcome/quality of life measured at the individual level

Figure 6 – Learning and Non-learning Cultures

a) A non learning organisation

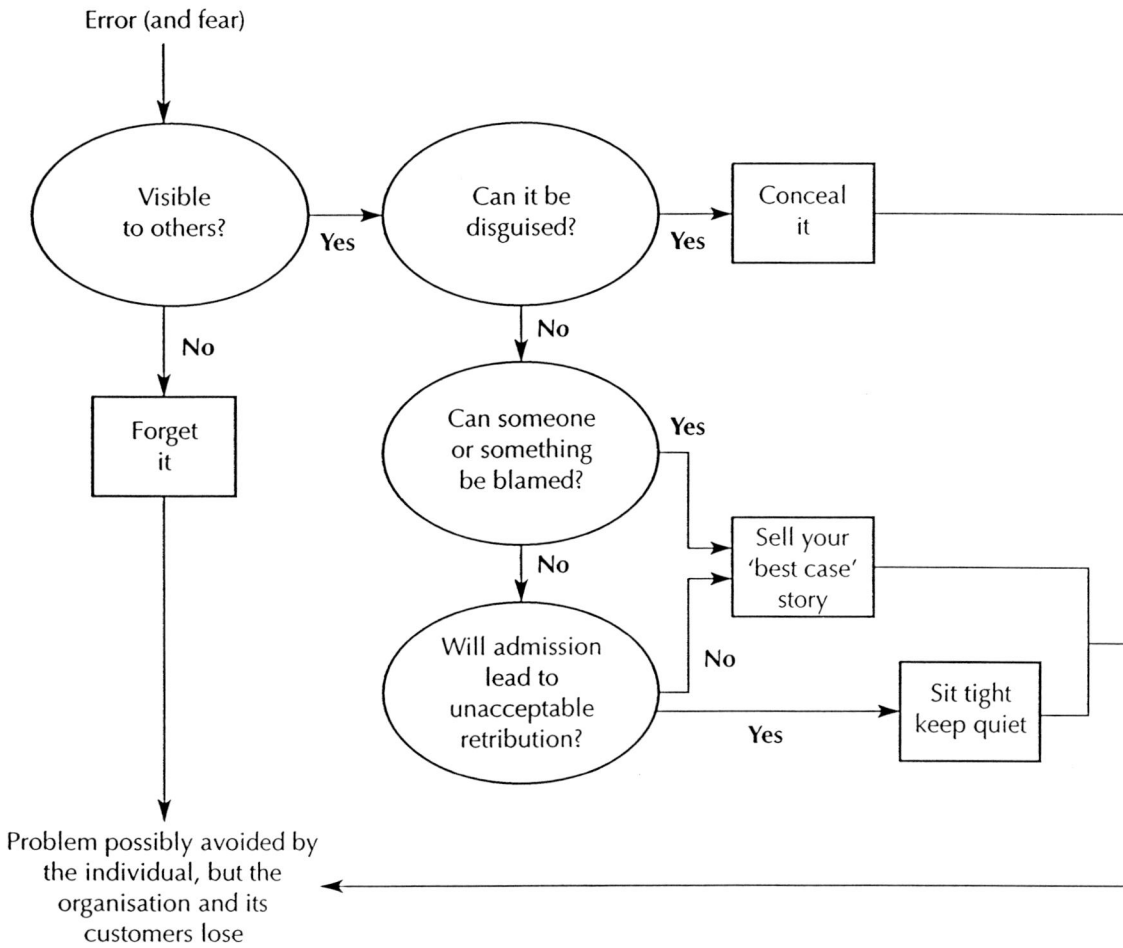

Error (and fear)

Visible to others? — Yes → Can it be disguised? — Yes → Conceal it

Visible to others? — No → Forget it

Can it be disguised? — No → Can someone or something be blamed?

Can someone or something be blamed? — Yes → Sell your 'best case' story

Can someone or something be blamed? — No → Will admission lead to unacceptable retribution?

Will admission lead to unacceptable retribution? — No → Sell your 'best case' story

Will admission lead to unacceptable retribution? — Yes → Sit tight keep quiet

Problem possibly avoided by the individual, but the organisation and its customers lose

b) A learning culture

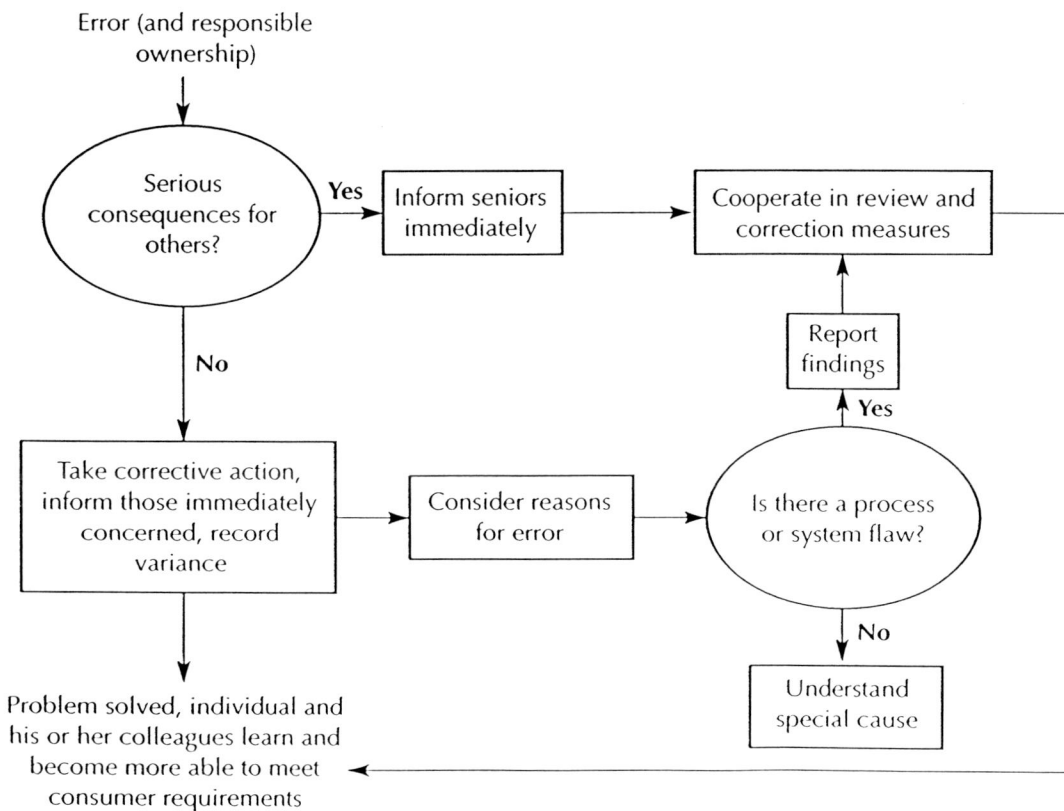

Error (and responsible ownership)

Serious consequences for others? — Yes → Inform seniors immediately → Cooperate in review and correction measures

Serious consequences for others? — No → Take corrective action, inform those immediately concerned, record variance → Consider reasons for error → Is there a process or system flaw?

Is there a process or system flaw? — Yes → Report findings → Cooperate in review and correction measures

Is there a process or system flaw? — No → Understand special cause

Problem solved, individual and his or her colleagues learn and become more able to meet consumer requirements

Figure 7 – Total Quality Management and the Inverted Status Pyramid

Traditional Management

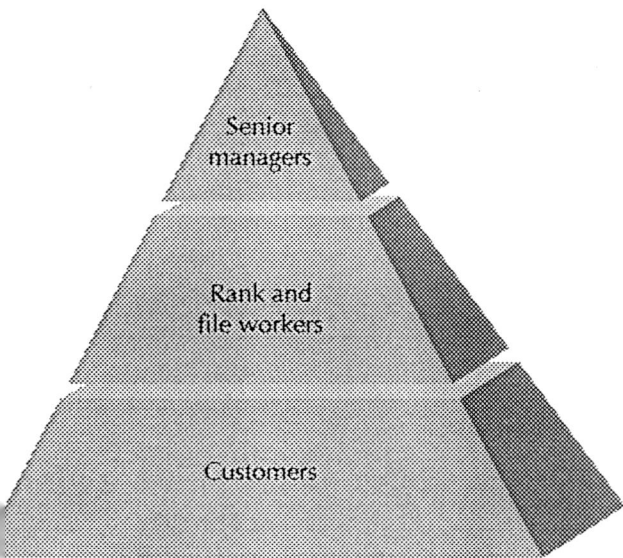

Senior managers

Rank and file workers

Customers

↑

Importance

Total Quality Management

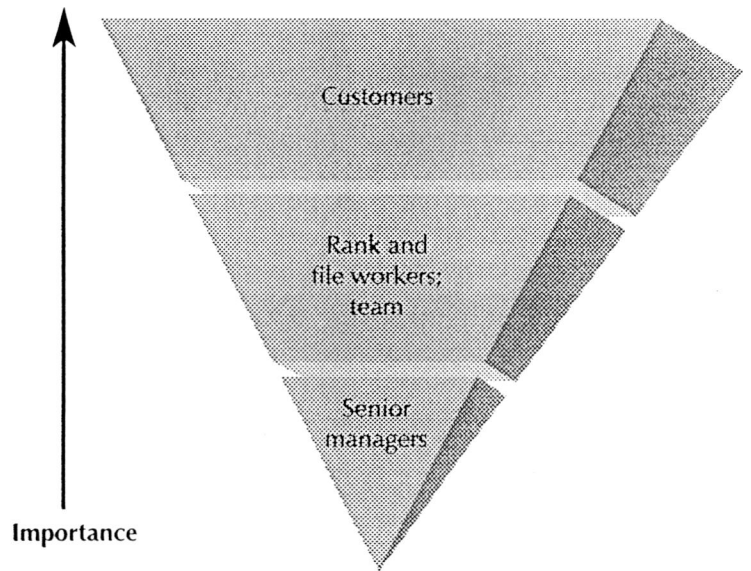

Customers

Rank and file workers; team

Senior managers

Figure 8 – Levels of Communication

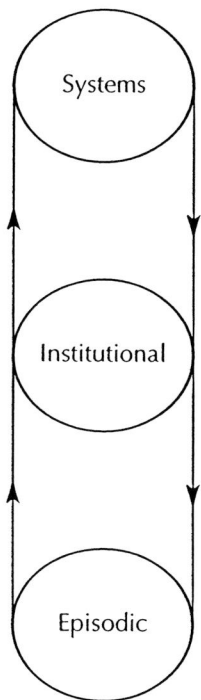

Systems

Institutional

Episodic

'Government and public affairs' contributions to national and local debates on broad public issues and interests, such as resource allocation priorities or the costs and benefits of alternative treatments. Presented via publications, media and group and individual meetings

'Public and customer relations' communications on specific matters relating to service developments and/or products, transmitted as appropriate via mass media, mailings and personal contacts

'Clinical communications' relating to the care and support of individuals and their families, conducted at a personal level